Juicing Your Way
To
Better Health

I0417512

Enjoy the Health Benefits
From Juicing Fruits and
Vegetables

RON KNESS

Contents

Disclaimer

This publication is for informational purposes only and is not intended as medical advice. Medical advice should always be obtained from a qualified medical professional for any health conditions or symptoms associated with them.

Every possible effort has been made in preparing and researching this material. We make no warranties with respect to the accuracy, applicability of its contents or any omissions.

See your healthcare professional before starting any diet or exercise program!

Get Started With Healthy Juicing

Whether it is just a fad or a trend that is here to stay, juicing is extremely popular among health conscious individuals. As more and more people experience the amazing results associated with this healthy lifestyle choice, its popularity is expected to grow.

Without question, juicing can be incorporated into your daily life to increase your overall health and vitality. By increasing your daily intake of healthy fruits and vegetables, you'll be giving your body the essential building blocks it needs. To get the most benefit out of juicing, you'll want to educate yourself on some of the basics before you get started. You'll find a wealth of information on these topics in the pages that follow.

The Benefits of Juicing at Home

If you are new to juicing, you may find the process to be a bit of a hassle. However, once you start to see and experience the many benefits associated with juicing, you may wonder how you ever got along without it. So commit to testing out your 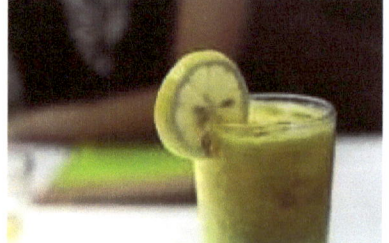 new lifestyle for at least several weeks before deciding if it is for you or not.

Important Tip: Making your own fresh juice drinks is better than buying ready-made juice products as they have to be treated and processed to extend shelf life. Therefore, homemade juices are fresher, plus you have more control over what you are putting into your body. And many of the ready-made juices contain a lot of sugar so if you are going to buy juice, be sure to read the label first.

When making your own homemade juices, however, it is important to consume the juice product as soon as it is ready. Exposure to air degrades the nutrients in your juice, so the sooner you drink it, the better.

It should also be noted that although fresh fruit juices are delicious and refreshing, be aware that many fruits are naturally high in sugar which can lead to unwanted weight gain and other unintended health issues. A better alternative is to combine complementary fruits and vegetables together to create healthy and delicious concoctions. Combining vegetable-based juices with a healthy balanced diet will help you achieve the results you desire.

Benefits of Healthy Juicing

One of the main benefits of juicing is that it is a lot easier to drink a single glass of nutrient-rich juice than it is to consume a comparable amount of whole fruits and vegetables. People are busy and most simply won't sit down and eat that much produce at one time. Instead, they'll reach for more convenient, but less healthy options.

Advantages of Juicing

There are many advantages associated with juicing. As
mentioned, juicing makes it easier to give your body the important nutrients, enzymes, vitamins and minerals it needs. In addition, some argue that juicing offers a more efficient way for your body to absorb 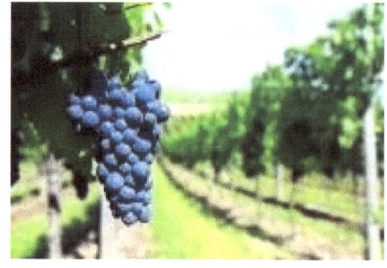 nutrients without placing undue pressure on your digestive system.

Juicing is also a great alternative for those who dislike vegetables and avoid eating them whenever possible. For these individuals, a glass of delicious juice lightly sweetened with a bit of pineapple or pear is a welcome alternative to a plate of steamed veggies.

There are tons of recipes available online to help you make delicious and creative juicing concoctions your whole family will love. When creating a collection of juice recipes you want to try, look for combinations that include both fruits and vegetables for the greatest health benefits.

Be aware that most juicing recipes include parts of the fruits and vegetables you would normally discard. With juicing, you'll often be advised to include leafy plant tops, rinds, skins, seeds and other parts that normally end up in the trash or compost pile. This is a real shame, because these items are often full of the essential nutrients your body needs.

When you start juicing, you will want to invest in a juicer

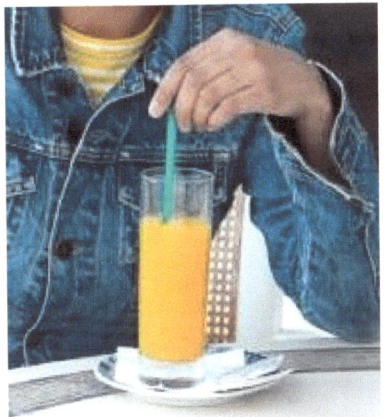

powerful enough to handle the types of fruits and vegetables you plan to use. This doesn't mean you have to break the bank or make a huge financial commitment to test out your new lifestyle. There are a number of really good entry-level centrifugal juicers on the market for around $50 or $60. These models don't offer all the bells and whistles of higher end units, but they are certainly worthy of your consideration.

Regardless of what kind of juicer you choose, consider it an investment in your long-term health. Making your own juices at home is infinitely better for you than picking up processed juices in your local grocery store. Those processed juices usually require some heating process to extend their shelf life, which can kill off valuable enzymes and nutrients. By making your own juice at home, you can keep the integrity of juice blends intact.

Healthy Juice Recipes

There are a lot of positive reasons to add juicing to your lifestyle. For starters, it is a very healthy way to lose weight and give your body the fuel it needs to thrive. When you take proper care of your body, you'll be amazed at how it rewards you with more energy and vitality than you've experienced in years.

Here are some delicious healthy juice recipes:

Lemony Apple:

- 2 apples

- 1 lemon

- 1" slice of ginger

This is a healthy remedy for colds as it is rich in flavonoid content. It also has a fresh and tangy taste that is quite invigorating.

Fresh OJ:
4 medium-sized oranges

Include as much of the white membranes as possible as it is rich in nutrients. Avoid using the whole peel as it can create an unpleasant taste and cause indigestion. Plus, you never want to juice the peel of any fruit that isn't organic.

Carrot-Apple Blend:

- 1 cup of spinach

- ½ cup of cucumber

- 2 stalks of celery including the leaves

- 3 carrots

- ½ medium apple

The skin of the dark green cucumber will provide the source of chlorophyll, which is a phytochemical that can help to build up the red blood cells. The cucumbers also contain silica, which is a mineral that is good for the skin.

A Very Berry Medley:

- 2 cups organic strawberries

- 2 cups organic blueberries

- 1.5 cups organic raspberries

It's important to use organic berries because their outer skins of so delicate and permeable. This delicious blend is an excellent source of antioxidants such as anthocyanins, flavonoid and ellagic acid, which are believed to offer anti-cancer and anti-heart disease benefits.

Pomegranate juice:

5 whole pomegranates – seeds only

Only the seeds are used in this recipe, while the pithy interior of the fruit and its outer rind are discarded. However, you may have better results using a blender to grind up the seeds. Then, strain the resulting liquid through cheesecloth and discard the remaining solids.

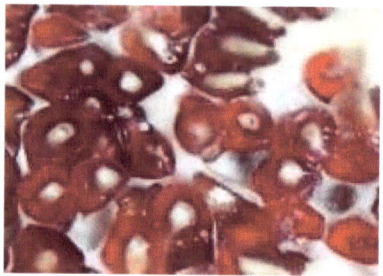

Juicing for Weight Loss

If done correctly, juicing can be an incredibly effective way to lose weight. However, most fruits contain a lot of natural sugar, which can make weight loss difficult. Therefore, you'll want to be sure to use juicing recipes that include lots of nutritious vegetables and only a little fruit for added sweetness, if weight loss is your primary goal.

Most juicing recipes that are designed for weight loss are very nutritious and satisfying. After all, if your weight loss-juicing regimen doesn't fill you up, you are more likely to reach for less healthy food choices to chase away those hunger pangs. You may have to experiment a bit to find combinations that work best for you, but that's half the fun of becoming a juicer!

When selecting ingredients for your juicing recipes, be sure to use fresh produce that has been cleaned thoroughly. Whenever possible, buy organic locally grown fruits and vegetables. Produce is at its healthiest when it is right off the plant. Buying locally grown 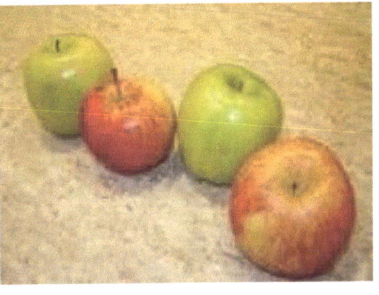 foods that are currently in season means it won't spend days in transit to your local grocery store. Although organic items cost more, taking that extra step will limit the amount of harmful chemicals and pesticides you consume.

Weight Loss Juicing Recipes:

Citrus Mint Juice:

- 1 grapefruit, peeled
  2 oranges, peeled
  20 stems lemon mint (use regular if you can't find the lemon variety)
  1 large seedless cucumber

Cucumber and Tomato Juice:

- 4 medium ripe tomatoes

- 2 medium seedless cucumbers

- 1 stalk celery with top

- ½ lime

- ¼ teaspoon cayenne pepper

Green Pineapple Juice:

- 1 cup fresh pineapple chunks, core and skin removed

- 5 stalks celery with tops

- 1" piece of ginger

- 1 large bunch kale leaves

Gingered Pear Juice:

- 1" piece of ginger root

- 2 large ripe pears, stems removed

- 1 large seedless cucumber, peeled

- 1 lime, peeled

- 1 bunch baby spinach

For all recipes, thoroughly wash and juice all ingredients. Serve immediately.

Wash and juice all ingredients. Season with salt and pepper, if desired.

Juicing for Kids

If you have kids, you already know getting them to eat enough fruits and vegetables can be a challenge. Perhaps you've already tried clever tricks to sneak in extra servings with their favorite meals. Fortunately, juicing is a great way to disguise healthy foods and make them look like a delicious treat instead.

It's true. Juicing can be a fun way to help your children get the extra vitamins and minerals their growing bodies need. The trick is to find juice combinations that are as delicious as they are nutritious. This is truly a win-win combination because your kids will think they're getting a yummy treat, and you'll be happy knowing they are finally consuming enough healthy fruits and veggies.

Depending on the age of your children and any underlying medical issues they may have, you will want to talk to their physician before making any drastic changes to their diet. Of course, a little moderation and common sense will go a long way as you start to adopt 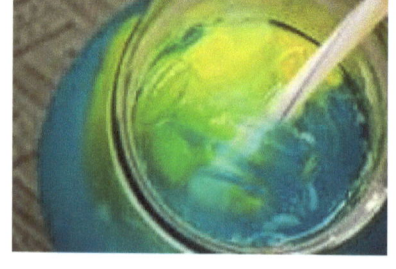 healthy lifestyle changes that work for your entire family.

Successful juicing with kids is really quite simple: Kids like stuff that tastes good. So when you first introduce juicing to your children, use fresh fruits and/or vegetables they already like. If they hate broccoli, don't assume they'll suddenly love it in liquid form.

Also, start out with simple juices made from one or two ingredients, rather than complex flavor combinations. This will allow your child to experience how delicious fresh juice can be, which will make them more likely to try other combinations in the future.

Then, once you've identified your child's favorite juices, use them as a base to create a variety of flavor combinations. Slowly add a small amount of other fruits or vegetables to further enhance the flavor profile and nutrient content of the juice.

Finally, many children love to experiment in the kitchen. Show them how the juicer works and allow them to see and experience the wonderful colors and flavors you can create with it. Letting them be part of the process and adding a little variety can go a long way toward raising lifelong juicing fans.

Here are a few simple juices and combos your children might enjoy:

- apple juice

- pineapple and carrot juice

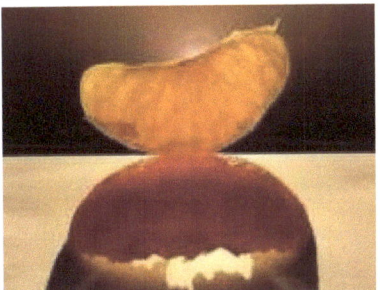

- orange juice

- orange and carrot juice

- pear juice

- apple and grape juice

Juicing for Anti-Aging

The better you take care of your body and give it what it needs to regenerate itself, the better you will look and feel in the long run. A healthy diet rich in vitamins and minerals is an important part of this equation. Juicing is a great way to get the valuable nutrients you need. As a result, it can help minimize the negative effects of the natural aging process.

Aging Gracefully

Juicing offers many health benefits because it can provide all the essential vitamins, minerals, amino acids, essential fatty acids, and enzymes your body needs to keep itself in peak form. The fruits, vegetables and leafy greens used in the juicing 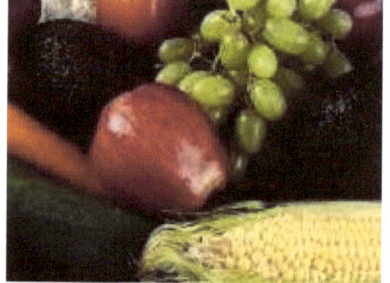 process are also packed with antioxidants and other substances that neutralize free radicals in your system, which helps counter-act the natural effects of aging.

Brightly colored fruits and vegetables are especially beneficial in your battle to age gracefully. Fruits such as oranges, cherries, tangerines, apples, blueberries, cranberries, melons, bananas, grapes, berries, kiwi, and mangoes are especially well known for their strong anti-aging properties. The best vegetables include carrots, squash, red and green cabbages, broccoli, and spinach as they offer great anti-aging benefits.

Don't be afraid to experiment a little to find your favorite flavor combinations. Once you find a good basic juice you really enjoy (e.g., apple and carrot), use it as a base to build upon for future recipes.

Anti-Aging Juicing Recipes

Apple Carrot Detox:

- 1 medium apple

- 1" chunk of fresh ginger

- 2 carrots

Apple-Berry Juice:

- 2 cups organic blueberries

- 2 medium apples

Beneficial Beet Juice

- ½ beet, washed and peeled

- 10 leaves fresh arugula

- 1 medium apple

- 1" fresh ginger root

- 1 whole lemon, peeled

For each recipe, thoroughly wash and juice all ingredients and serve immediately.

Juicing for Detoxification

When your body is full of toxins, it is unable to properly absorb the valuable nutrients found in the foods you eat. This can lead to an unhealthy balance where your body is literally "starved" for the building materials it needs. Juicing is a great way to detoxify your body and improve the way your body absorbs enzymes, vitamins and minerals. The result is a stronger immune system and higher energy levels.

As previously noted, consuming nutrient-rich juice made from organic fruits and vegetables gives your body the tools it needs to operate efficiently. Your lungs, kidneys, liver, skin and digestive system all play an important role in helping your body eliminate waste material and unwanted toxins from your body. The better nutrition you provide for 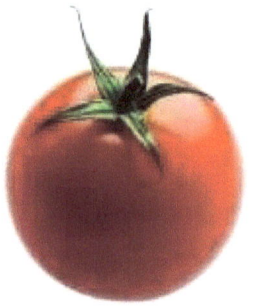 your body, the easier it will be for your organs and systems to do their job and "flush out" the toxins that have accumulated over time.

As an added bonus, some people who follow a detoxifying juicing regimen claim they no longer have cravings for processed or artificially sweetened foods, which makes it much easier to stick to a healthy diet long term.

Ideal juicing ingredients for detoxification include lettuce, dark green kale, carrots, beet greens, cilantro, parsley, celery sticks, collard greens, endive, spinach, dandelion greens, purple and green cabbage, and lemons.

Detox Juicing Recipes:

Blackberry Beet Juice

- 12 oz. organic blackberries

- 1" piece fresh ginger

- 2 medium beets with tops

- 3 medium apples

Green Detox Blend:

- 8 stalks celery with tops

- 1" piece fresh ginger

- 1 handful fresh baby spinach leaves

- 1 medium green apple

- 20 stems fresh parsley leaves

- 1 lime, peeled

- 1 lemon, peeled

For each recipe, thoroughly wash and juice all ingredients and serve immediately.

Juicing for Disease Prevention

By now, we've established that juicing can be an integral part of healthy lifestyle. Giving your body the building blocks it needs to function at peak efficiency can help you enjoy a healthier, longer life free from the complications of chronic or life-threatening diseases. Juicing is an easy and cost-effective way to provide the nutrients your body needs to accomplish this.

There are many recommended juicing combinations that claim to help your body fight off disease. For example, beets (aka beetroot) are very popular in juicing recipes aimed at preventing disease. They are believed to dramatically reduce the risks of heart disease, strokes, Alzheimer's and dementia. The bright red juice contains key nutrients, which can also help reduce blood pressure.

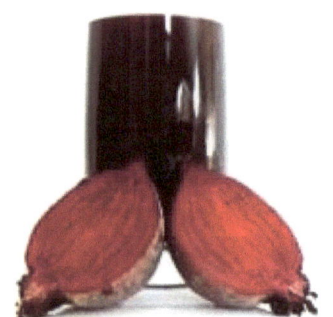

Pomegranates are considered another disease-fighting juicing ingredient thought to lower cardiovascular risks. In addition, tomato juice combinations may help reduce the risk of heart disease and control diabetic symptoms, as well. Tomato juice can also reduce the risk of developing life-threatening diseases such as cancer and coronary heart disease. This claim is based on the high level of lycopene found in fresh tomatoes.

Additional ingredients that can be used to help prevent disease include broccoli, Brussels sprouts, butternut squash, cabbage, Chinese broccoli, kale, spinach, parsley, collards greens, mustards green, Swiss chard, beetroot, carrots, cauliflower, cucumber, green pepper, sweet potatoes, lettuce and celery. Look for juicing recipes featuring these ingredients for the best results.

Again, these recommendations aren't meant to replace qualified medical advice, but instead are to be used as guidelines to help you establish a healthy, well-rounded diet. A diet based on organic, locally grown fruits and vegetables is a great foundation for achieving the healthy lifestyle you want and deserve.

Choosing the Perfect Centrifugal Juicer for a Healthier Lifestyle

In the inspiring true story "**Fat, Sick & Nearly Dead**," Australian businessman Joe Cross transforms his life by following an intensive 60-day juicing-only program. Along the way, he sheds an impressive 82 pounds and frees himself from a debilitating autoimmune disease. Most importantly, after following this 60-day juicing regimen, all of his key health indicators showed that he was healthier than he had been since he was a child. You can learn his story from his DVD on Amazon at: http://amzn.to/2cyKG9w.

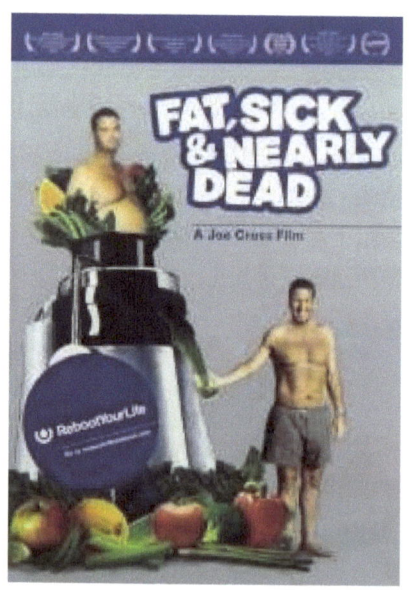

Clearly, juicing offers many wonderful health benefits. It can help burn fat, regulate your blood pressure, firm your skin, improve your memory, and give you more energy. Whether you plan to add juicing to your everyday lifestyle or are planning to adopt an intensive short-term "reboot" juicing regimen, your digestive system and body will thank you for it.

A healthy diet is the key to a healthy lifestyle. By extracting the nutrients, enzymes, vitamins and minerals found in whole fruits and vegetables, a centrifugal juicer can put you on the road to feeling and looking better than you have in years.

These units are perfect if you are just getting started juicing or if you have a limited-to-moderate budget. However, just because these affordable machines cost less than their masticating counterparts does not mean you'll be short changed in terms of quality and value.

How Centrifugal Juicers Work

There are two main types of juicers: centrifugal and masticating. As the name suggests, centrifugal juicers uses centrifugal (moving away from the center) force to extract liquids from fruits, vegetables and leafy greens.

Operating at very high speeds of anywhere from 2,000 to 14,000 revolutions per minute (RPM), centrifugal juicers use an incredible amount of force to separate the juice from the pulp in the foods you are juicing. In terms of composition, these juicers normally feature a feed tube on top where you can add your produce to the unit. Plus, they employ some type of filter to catch the pulp while the juice goes into your glass or a receptive container.

As opposed to masticating juicers, centrifugal juicing machines are less expensive, work faster, and offer easier clean up. These qualities make centrifugal juicers very popular among first-time juicers and those on a limited budget. However, with over 240 centrifugal models to choose from on Amazon, it can be hard to decide which one is right for you.

Since all centrifugal juicers work basically the same way, you need to decide how much you are willing to spend and what features are most important to you. In terms of budget, you can pick up a decent entry-level unit for around $50 or $60 brand new. If you want to try juicing without making a large cash investment, the **Stainless Steel Hamilton Beach 67608 Big Mouth Juice Extractor** on Amazon at: http://amzn.to/2cm7mKY is worth a closer look.

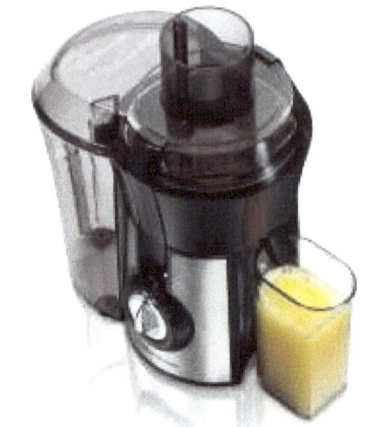

On the other hand, if you want a very high-end centrifugal juicer with all the bells and whistles, prepare to spend hundreds or even thousands of dollars for a commercial-grade appliance suitable for home use. There are also a ton of great options in the middle of these two extremes that provide outstanding value for approximately $100 to $150.

Once you've established your budget, decide which features are most important to you. For example, if you have a small kitchen with limited counter or storage space, you may want a compact unit with a small overall footprint. If you don't want to spend a lot of time chopping fruits and vegetables prior to juicing, look for a model with a large feeding tube. You'll also want to consider construction materials, like durable stainless steel blades or BPA-free plastic parts, before making your decision.

Fortunately, with the popularity of online shopping sites like Amazon, it is easy to get feedback from others who have purchased and used the centrifugal juicing models you are considering.

Look for units with above a 4.0 overall rating from a decent number of reviewers to get a good idea of the pros and cons of each unit.

Don't get too bogged down in the details, though. Make an informed decision based on the above-noted criteria and take the plunge. Before you know it, your new centrifugal juicer will help you achieve a much healthier lifestyle.

Why Masticating Juicers Make the Most Sense ... and Juice

If you are in the market for a new juicer, you'll soon realize there are two main types of machines available: centrifugal and masticating. There are numerous pros and cons associated with each type of unit. In general, centrifugal units cost less, are easier to clean and operate faster than masticating units. However, masticating juicers offer quieter operation and are a lot more efficient in terms of extracting every last drop of juice from the fruits and vegetables you buy. Over time, a good masticating juicer can help pay for itself by cutting your grocery costs.

Masticating juicers get their name from the word masticate, which means "to chew." These juicing models work by utilizing a screw-like auger mechanism to slowly grind the fruits and vegetables you feed into them. This process is what makes masticating juicers extremely efficient and a lot less noisy compared to centrifugal juicers.

As a rule, you will invest more upfront for a quality masticating juicer than you would for a centrifugal unit. In exchange, you'll be rewarded with higher juice yields from every piece of produce you put into it and a much quieter operation. In addition, masticating units offer a number of other advantages worth considering.

For starters, many of the most popular and healthiest juicing recipes involve leafy greens and wheat grass. Most centrifugal juicers simply are not able to transform these items into very much juice.

Without question, you'll get a much higher juice yield when dealing juicing nutrient-rich foods like kale, cabbage, wheat grass and spinach with a masticating juicer.

In addition, masticating juicers incorporate a lot less oxygen into your juice than centrifugal machines. This translates into a more deeply colored and richly flavored end product. Plus, this also allows you to store your healthy juice creations in your refrigerator for up to three full days. With centrifugal juicers, it is recommended you drink the juices you create within 24 hours. As an added bonus, less air in your juice can mean less bloating and unpleasant gas for you.

So even though you'll typically invest more in a masticating juicer up front, less oxygen in your juice means your juice will last longer and taste better. You'll also receive the maximum amount of juice possible from the vegetables, fruits and leafy greens that you use. Plus, if you need to use your juicer late at night or early in the morning, a masticating machine won't disturb other members of your household.

You can also count on even the most affordable masticating juicer to be a durable and lasting investment. That is nice, because you probably want to benefit from the amazing health benefits juicing can offer for an extended period of time. High-quality masticating juicers can provide years of efficient and quiet operation with minimal upkeep on your part. Fashionable stainless steel construction and other attractive design features also make them stylish accessories for your kitchen.

Fortunately, you can find high quality, highly rated masticating units with attractive price tags. In fact, some features that are considered "basic" on masticating units are marketed as high-end and expensive upgrades on centrifugal juicers. In some cases, you can find masticating models that require a smaller investment than less efficient centrifugal units.

In other words, it pays to do your homework first. If you have decided a full-featured and extremely efficient, quiet masticating juicer is perfect for you and your family, it's time to choose the right one. With so many options available, narrowing it down to just one can be a little confusing.

As with any significant purchase, personal preference is important when making this decision. So you'll want to determine your budget and what features are most important to you before making a decision. Once you know what your "must haves" are – and what you can live without – finding the perfect masticating juicer will be a lot easier!

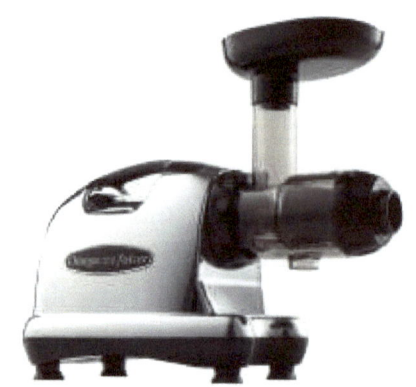

If I can recommend one juicer, the Omega J8006 is a great one to buy. You can find it on Amazon at: http://amzn.to/2cyM4Jg.

50 Tips to Juice Like a Pro

1. Make a commitment to juicing and stick to it, this can be tricky if you are not used to the practice but with time, dedication and regular use it can become so deeply embedded that it will simply be something you won't want to live without. It can take several weeks to form a solid juicing habit, so stick with it and make sure to juice regularly.

2. Create a juicing schedule. Make plans depending on how much your juicer can juice at one time, how much prep is necessary for produce, and how much time you can dedicate each day or every other day to be sure that you have fresh juice available at all times.

3. Stick with a regular juicing schedule to support the habit – the good habit. Studies show that consumption of large doses of specific vitamins, minerals, and enzymes can aid in the prevention and management of symptoms associated with heart disease, cancer, and strokes and can strengthen immunity against colds and flu, increase bone density and improve the condition of the skin. We know that studies have shown that it is recommended that we consume six to eight servings of vegetables and fruits daily. This can be challenging for many people, but juicing ensures that you reach the recommended daily intake for vegetables in a convenient manner.

4. Buy a quality juicer - many vegetables, like beets and carrots, are actually quite difficult to pulverize properly, and cheap juicers will not do the job. Buying a juicer that is powerful enough to pulverize efficiently and rapidly is one of the keys to buying a great juicer. If you plan to juice a lot of hard vegetables, your best choice is a centrifugal juicer.

5. If you plan to juice mostly greens, then consider a masticating juicer that is great for softer greens and also supplies a high juice yield.

6. Consider the size of the mixing container. If you go too small, you'll only be able to juice a little at a time, so make sure you invest in a unit that has the capacity for your juicing needs. This is especially important for large families.

7. Keep a produce shopping list to stay organized and have all the ingredients you need at hand when you want to juice.

8. If you plan to juice in the morning then prep your produce as needed the night before. This is especially useful when your mornings are rushed or time limited.

9. Always wash produce thoroughly to eliminate all dirt particles, and some of the pesticides when not buying organic produce. This is especially important with leafy greens where dirt hides between the leaves.

10. Line your juicer's pulp basket with a plastic bag for easy clean up.

11. Juice every day to build a healthy habit. When daily juicing is not possible, you can store juice in the fridge in an airtight container for up to 3 days.

12. Juice vegetables that you do not normally eat. Every vegetable provides a different benefit to the body but everyone is different in terms of what vegetables they enjoy eating, and so they skip those they don't like due to either taste, smell or texture. Juicing these allows you to obtain benefits from vegetables that you would not ordinarily consume, and since you can mask their taste with fruit, lemons, ginger and other enhancers getting these nutrients becomes much less of a burden.

13. Consider sugar content of fruits when you juice, as some have so much sugar they should be consumed in moderation or avoided altogether, especially for those who need to avoid spikes in blood sugar levels (diabetics), those with weight issues, and definitely those who are juicing for weight loss.

14. Taste as you go and adjust accordingly, just as you would during cooking.

15. Consuming juices first thing in the morning or at any time when your stomach is empty will optimize the rate at which the vitamins, minerals, antioxidants, and enzymes are absorbed and used by the body.

It also gives you a great energy boost to kick-start your day with the drive you need. Additionally, consuming raw fruit and vegetables provides an intensive boost of vitamins and enzymes, which are directed straight to the blood stream. This means that your digestive system does not need to process the fruit and vegetables as they would if you were to consume them whole.

16. Juice high water vegetables, like cucumbers and broccoli. People often struggle with reaching the recommended daily intake of water. With six to eight glasses being the goal, some find it difficult to reach this intake. Many juicing combinations incorporate an element of water as the basis for the recipe, and indeed many vegetables and fruits have a high water concentration, meaning that you are extracting water during the juicing process. Juicing provides a great strategy for increasing your water intake each day to hydrate your body.

17. Make sure to juice vegetables with fruit. If you only consume fruit-based juices, your intake of sugar and calories will be unnecessarily high. By integrating vegetable juicing into your daily diet, you will be able to optimize the volume of vitamins, minerals, antioxidants, and enzymes being absorbed by your body.

18. Make sure that you follow the 80/20 rule when it comes to the ratio of vegetables to fruit. 80% vegetables that will give you the immunity, wellness, and energy boost you need and 20% fruit for more nutrients and taste. So, add an apple to give some sweetness or an orange if you crave some zesty citrus flavor.

19. Make sure that you include one or two root vegetables in your juicing combination. By adding in a carrot or beet into your recipe, you will be able to give the juice an intense boost of antioxidants, while also gaining a sweet but earthy flavor, which makes it more palatable when drinking.

20. To optimize the nutritional properties of your juice you need to ensure that you include a minimum of at least, one leafy green vegetable such as kale, broccoli, or chard, which will give you an enormous amount of unique nutrients.

21. High water content vegetables such as a cucumbers or celery will assist in diffusing the very (and sometimes overpowering) flavors of kale, broccoli, or chard, which help to ensure that the juice you prepare is easy to drink.

22. Add some kind of garnish to not only provide a concentrated and intensive vitamin boost but also to make the juice really tasty. Great options include, ginger, lemons, limes or mint.

23. Re-juice any still wet pulp to get the most bang for your juicing buck.

24. Juice to improve the aging process - as we age our ability to digest what we need can become impaired as our organs work less optimally. By preparing food in this liquid and raw form, it becomes "pre-digested" which means that the body can absorb the vitamins, minerals, antioxidants and enzymes quickly and most efficiently.

25. Juicing fruit alone greatly increases your sugar intake, which can lead to weight gain and erratic blood sugar spikes that actually stimulate hunger, negating the positive benefits that juicing offers.

26. Include lots of vegetables in your juicing to benefit from chlorophyll, which is a compound that acts as the life force within the plant. This compound also offers significant beneficial properties for humans. Consumed raw as part of a juicing regime, the chlorophyll is digested straight into your bloodstream meaning that you are getting all of the benefits that the vegetables have to offer. Wheatgrass has the highest amount of chlorophyll.

27. Drink more green juice. Green juice is juice made mostly from dark leafy greens, such as kale, broccoli, and spinach, but can also include celery, cabbage, broccoli, and apples. Green juice is your best choice in a highly nutrient rich and low sugar drink.

28. For some, the perception that green colored juice looks bad and therefore tastes bad can interfere with the healthy practice of juicing. You can get past your perceived dislike for the color of the juice by adding in some red berries or orange carrots that will improve the color and taste to get a boost of vitamins, minerals, antioxidants and enzymes that you need to optimize your mental and physical health and wellbeing.

29. To help you become acclimated to the taste of vegetable juice, ease yourself into the taste of green vegetable-based juices so that you aren't immediately repelled and become turned off juicing forever. Start with mild-tasting vegetables such as celery and cucumbers. As you start to build your juicing palette, you can start to incorporate lettuce, kale, spinach, parsley, or cilantro.

30. To counteract that bitterness of vegetable and green juices, you can add in elements of lemon or lime, grapefruits, cranberries or ginger, each of which have excellent properties that are associated with health and wellbeing.

31. Continue to eat whole vegetables and fruits even while juicing as they produce important insoluble fiber that your body needs.

32. It is best to consume juice on an empty stomach. This will give your body an optimum energy boost and allow for optimal digestion of all of the vitamins, minerals, antioxidants and enzymes that you need to go about your day.

33. Engage the whole family in juicing, as this is a great way to increase vegetable intake in young kids who hate eating them to make sure they benefit from the regular consumption of vitamins, minerals, antioxidants, and enzymes.

34. Collect juicing recipes, but also create your own blends to find combinations that please your palate and allow you to remain positive about your new habit.

35. To improve the health and vitality of your skin try combining cucumbers and a small apple (for taste).

36. To fight aging, choose a juicing combination that includes water/milk/aloe-vera juice, blueberries, strawberries, kale, and beetroot.

37. To enhance your libido you can combine coconut water, celery, banana, ginger, basil, and figs.

38. To give yourself an energy boost juice a combination that includes cucumbers, celery, kale, spinach, parsley, lemon and ginger.

39. To satisfy your sweet tooth juice a combination that includes apples, celery, and stir in a little cinnamon.

40. To boost your immune system and prevent the cold and flu, juice blends that include beetroot, carrots, celery, broccoli, garlic, ginger, lemon, and cayenne pepper.

41. If you are overworked or feeling the effects of stress in your life, prepare a stress relief juice with spinach, broccoli, celery, and carrots.

42. If you want to improve your gut health and digestion, boost your intake of papain, which is an enzyme found in papaya that helps digest proteins. Try a juice that includes papaya, kale, cabbage, ginger, and lemon.

43. Juice organic produce - Use only organic vegetables to avoid toxins, and to increase the nutritional value of your produce and healthy enzyme intake.

44. Enhance your juices with ground nuts and seeds and protein powders.
Adding protein powder to your juice makes for a great meal replacement juice.

45. Beware of long term juice cleanses, and make sure to ask your doctor before starting any sort of juice fast.

46. Engage your kids in the juicing process. Let them pick out their own ingredients to get them excited about fruits and vegetables.

47. Buy an airtight container so you can refrigerate your juice and also take it with you to work, the gym or while running errands.

48. If you have an adversity to the taste of vegetable juice, don't worry, for many it is an acquired taste. Once your body starts to feel the health benefits you'll be hooked.

49. Balance high yield produce like celery, tomatoes, apples, and cucumbers, with a low yield vegetable like kale to get more juice in your glass.

50. Use herbs and spices in your juice, including basil, parsley, cilantro, mint, turmeric, cumin, nutmeg, ginger and hot peppers to not only enhance flavor but to get their numerous health benefits.

Other Juicing Books by This Author

If you would like to read more about juicing, here is a list of the titles, CreateSpace links and descriptions:

Fight Cancer With Juicing
https://www.createspace.com/6155567

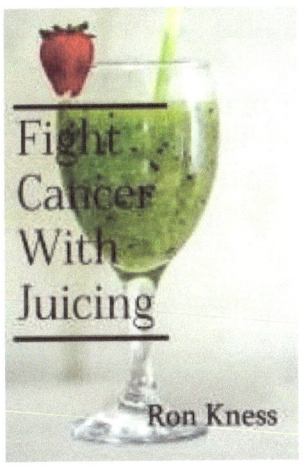

Juicing is a healthy practice that has allowed millions of people to boost their nutrition. Juicing fruits and vegetables provides you important antioxidants, which scavenge for oxygen free radicals that can damage cellular structures, including DNA. When DNA is damaged, it can result in mutations that lead to cancer.

Well-balanced nutrition from a variety of healthy whole foods helps support and maintain on-going good health, and experts agree that nutrition plays a key role in preventing chronic and terminal illness.

When juicing is done right, that is when the majority of your juice blends is comprised of vegetables and very low sugar fruit, you can easily boost your nutritional intake thereby improving your health and lower your risks for cancer.

This book gives you the information needed to not only help prevent cancer in the first place, but to help fight it naturally if you already have it.

Juicing for Health: The Complete Guide to Juicing for Good Nutrition

https://www.createspace.com/6241849

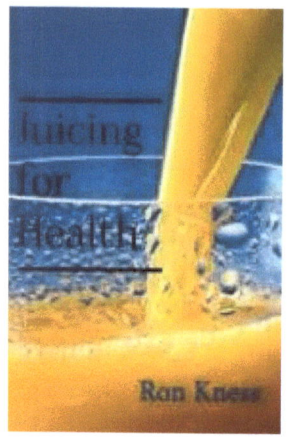

It's well documented that many of us need to increase our daily intake of fruit and vegetables. We are the champions of the world when it comes to getting enough of the macronutrients carbs, protein, and fat, but we're sorely lacking when it comes to getting more micronutrients.

While the Centers For Disease Control recommend adults consume about 1 ½ to 2 cups of fruit and 2 to 3 cups of vegetables daily, an analysis of American diets between 2007 and 2010 found that 50% of the population ate less than 1 cup of fruit and less than 1 ½ cups of vegetables.

An astounding 76% of people did not eat nearly enough fruit, and 87% did not eat enough vegetables.

Many people simply don't like eating vegetables. Broccoli is tough, cabbage is chewy, and carrots can break your teeth if they haven't been boiled long enough and let's not get started on that stringy asparagus!

However, fruit and vegetables are where essential micronutrients are to be found and juicing is a great way to easily pack more of them into a well-balanced and healthy diet.

Thousands have joined the juicing revolution and for good reason, it is healthy, convenient and allows you to get key vitamins and minerals from plant foods that may be missing from your diet.

About the Author

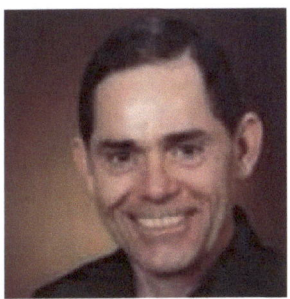

I grew up in Central Minnesota, where my parents owned and operated a fishing resort. Once out of high school I tried a couple of semesters of college, only to quit halfway through the Spring term; I decided at that time that college wasn't for me.

Then I decided to follow my father's previous occupation as an auto mechanic. I graduated from a two-year of vocational training course and worked as a mechanic for five years. While in vocational training, I decided to join the National Guard where I eventually ended up working full-time for 32 years.

So how does all of this relate to writing? In one of my leadership schools, the instructor, who was an English teacher at a juvenile detention center, presented writing to me in a whole new way - a way that started to develop my interest in working with words.

I eventually went back to college on the GI Bill while I was working and earned my Bachelor's degree in Business Administration.

Taking a class or two per semester at night and on weekends took me seven years to complete my degree.

Fast forward about 40 years and I now have published over 75 books on Amazon for Kindle, CreateSpace and other publishing platforms.

Besides my own writing, I also ghostwrite ebooks, reports, articles, blogs and do Kindle conversions for clients on a variety of topics.

Today my wife and I are retired from our careers and live in Gold Canyon, AZ. I now write as a retirement business where you'll find me happily sitting in my office typing away on my laptop as I work on my next book or ghostwriting project . . . that is if we are not traveling on a cruise ship - our new-found mode of travel.

www.ingramcontent.com/pod-product-compliance
Lightning Source LLC
Chambersburg PA
CBHW050841290526
45792CB00001B/483